COMPLETE GUIDE TO UNDERSTANDING TOTAL JOINT REPLACEMENT

Essential Insights For Recovery Tips, Pain Management, And Post-Surgery Exercises

KLEIN HOYLE

Disclaimer

The content in this book is based on the author's expertise and comprehension of the topic. The author has no affiliation or link with any corporation, business, or person. This book is meant to give general information and educational material only, and it should not be interpreted as professional medical advice. Always seek the advice of a skilled healthcare expert if you have any queries about medical issues or treatments. The author and publisher expressly disclaim any responsibility resulting directly or indirectly from the use or use of the information included in this book.

Table of Contents

ABOUT THIS BOOK

The "Complete Guide to Understanding Total Joint Replacement" is a crucial resource for anybody considering joint replacement surgery or who wants to learn more about this groundbreaking medical treatment. This thorough book starts with an overview of total joint replacement, describing its importance and the many kinds of joints that may be replaced. It also offers an intriguing review of the history and progress of joint replacement surgery, laying the groundwork for a more in-depth knowledge of this medical accomplishment.

This book investigates the origins and symptoms of joint degeneration, stressing the need for early detection. Readers will learn how joint deterioration may affect everyday living, emphasizing the need for immediate medical care. This section explains why knowing joint health is important and how it may impact one's quality of life.

Preparation for complete joint replacement is thoroughly discussed, with practical guidance on first consultations, medical testing, and assessments. It also discusses the essential lifestyle changes, as well as the mental and emotional preparations needed before surgery. This instruction is helpful for patients who want to go into surgery with confidence and a thorough knowledge of the procedure.

This book then divides joint replacement surgery into four categories: knee, hip, shoulder, and elbow. Each kind is explored in depth, giving readers a complete grasp of the various techniques and their distinct concerns. This category serves to demystify procedures, making information more accessible and thorough.

A thorough discussion of the surgical process follows, including anesthetic choices, surgical methods, possible risks and consequences, and predicted results. This part is critical for establishing realistic expectations and assisting patients in preparing for their operation and early postoperative care.

Recovery is another essential topic, including information on hospital stays, postoperative care, pain management, physical therapy, and rehabilitation. This part walks patients through the gradual return to everyday activities, stressing the significance of each recovery phase for best results.

Managing expectations after surgery is also fully discussed. Readers are informed about reasonable expectations, normal healing problems, and the long-term advantages of joint replacement. This book also provides lifestyle recommendations for preserving joint health, ensuring that patients are well-informed about life following surgery.

This book addresses probable consequences by outlining measures for infection prevention, blood clot prevention, and coping with implant failure. It also addresses revision procedures and the psychological assistance required to deal with difficulties, offering a comprehensive approach to patient care.

Living with joint replacements is thoroughly discussed, with an emphasis on preserving joint health after surgery via frequent check-ups, physical activities, and exercises. Tips for avoiding future joint issues are also offered, allowing patients to live a healthy and active lifestyle with their new joints.

Finally, This book discusses potential advancements and improvements in joint replacement technology and materials. Emerging surgical procedures and advances in regenerative medicine are explored, providing insight into the future of joint replacement surgery and its potential to improve patient outcomes.

This book is an invaluable resource for anybody seeking to comprehend the entire breadth of joint replacement surgery, from the early decision-making process to living with a joint replacement and the bright future of this medical specialty.

CHAPTER 1

Introduction To Total Joint Replacement

What Is Total Joint Replacement?

Total joint replacement, also known as arthroplasty, is a surgical operation in which a damaged or arthritic joint is removed and replaced with a prosthesis composed of metal, ceramic, or plastic materials. The goal of this procedure is to reduce pain and restore joint function, enabling patients to resume normal activities with better mobility and quality of life.

During the operation, the surgeon removes the diseased or damaged components of the joint and replaces them with artificial elements that move and function like a normal joint. The prosthetic joint is intended to mirror natural movement and alignment, resulting in a stable and pain-free range of motion. This operation is most typically done on weight-bearing joints such as the hips and knees, but it may also be used on the shoulders, elbows, wrists, and ankles.

Why Is It Needed?

Individuals with significant joint pain and impairment caused by illnesses such as osteoarthritis, rheumatoid arthritis, post-traumatic arthritis, or avascular necrosis are usually advised to undergo total joint replacement. These disorders may cause considerable degradation of joint cartilage, resulting in discomfort, stiffness, and impaired function.

Osteoarthritis, the most prevalent cause of joint replacement, is a degenerative condition in which cartilage breaks down, resulting in bone-on-bone contact and painful mobility. Rheumatoid arthritis, an autoimmune illness, generates persistent inflammation, which may harm joint cartilage and surrounding tissues. Post-traumatic arthritis develops as a result of a joint injury, while avascular necrosis occurs when the blood supply to the bone is disturbed, leading bone tissue to die.

When conservative therapies including medication, physical therapy, and lifestyle changes fail to relieve symptoms, complete joint replacement becomes a possibility. The objective is to alleviate pain, improve joint function, and improve overall quality of life for patients who have exhausted all other therapy choices.

Types Of Joints That Can Be Replaced

Several joints in the human body are suitable for complete joint replacement, with the hip and knee being the most typically replaced. However, advances in medical technology have made it feasible to replace additional joints.

• Hip replacement involves replacing the ball-and-socket joint with a prosthetic ball, stem, and cup.

• Knee replacement involves resurfacing damaged cartilage with metal and plastic components.

• Shoulder Replacement: Artificial components are used to replace the upper arm bone's ball and shoulder blade socket.

• Elbow Replacement: Replaces humerus and ulna bones with a hinge-like prosthetic.

• Prosthetics are used to replace injured ankle joint surfaces.

• Wrist Replacement: Replace broken wrist joints with metal and plastic components.

Each form of joint replacement is designed to meet the unique anatomical and functional needs of the joint being replaced, to restore as much natural mobility as possible.

Brief History And Evolution Of Joint Replacement Surgery

The history of joint replacement surgery goes back to the late nineteenth and early twentieth century's, with early efforts focused on partial replacements and interposition arthroplasty, in which foreign materials were put between joint surfaces to relieve discomfort. These early operations had a low success rate and a considerable risk of complications.

The contemporary age of joint replacement started in the 1960s, with the advancement of new materials and surgical procedures. Sir John Charnley, a British orthopedic surgeon, is credited with performing the first successful complete hip replacement. He invented the idea of employing a metal ball with a polyethylene socket, which greatly improved results and durability. Charnley's low-friction arthroplasty established the gold standard for hip replacements and paved the way for subsequent improvements.

Since then, joint replacement surgery has been constantly refined and improved. Advances in biomaterials, such as titanium and sophisticated ceramics, have improved prosthetic joint lifetime and function. Minimally invasive surgical procedures and computer-assisted navigation have increased implant placement accuracy, resulting in better results and quicker recovery periods.

Today, joint replacement surgery is one of the most successful and widely done orthopedic operations, with millions of individuals benefitting from increased pain alleviation and mobility. Ongoing research and development continue to drive innovation in this sector, with the promise of even better outcomes for future patients.

CHAPTER 2

Understanding Joint Degeneration

Causes Of Joint Degeneration

Joint degeneration, which may lead to disorders like osteoarthritis, is caused by the slow loss of cartilage—the smooth tissue that covers the ends of bones in a joint. Several things may impact this breakdown.

1. Age: As we age, the accumulated wear and strain on our joints hastens cartilage breakdown. The body's capacity to repair and replace cartilage declines, increasing susceptibility to joint deterioration.

2. Genetics: Family history contributes significantly to the risk of joint deterioration. Certain genetic markers and hereditary disorders may raise the risk of getting osteoarthritis and other degenerative joint illnesses.

3. Obesity: Excess body weight increases stress on weight-bearing joints such as the knees and hips. This additional pressure may accelerate the wear and tear on cartilage, resulting in faster deterioration.

4. Joint Injuries: Previous injuries, such as fractures or ligament tears, may damage cartilage or change joint mechanics, making it more prone to deterioration over time. Repetitive stress from sports or physically demanding employment may also lead to joint degeneration.

5. Overuse: Repetitive motions or overuse of certain joints, as observed in athletes or people with physically demanding employment, may hasten cartilage deterioration. This is particularly true for joints subjected to regular high-impact exercises.

6. Chronic inflammation caused by illnesses such as rheumatoid arthritis may destroy the cartilage and underlying bone, resulting in joint deterioration. Inflammatory processes produce enzymes and substances that destroy joint tissues.

Symptoms And Signs Of Joint Degeneration

Recognizing the symptoms and indicators of joint degeneration is critical for early detection and treatment. Common indications are:

1. The most common symptom is joint pain, which may vary from mild aching to severe agony. Pain often intensifies with activity and diminishes with rest, but in late stages, it might last even during times of inactivity.

2. **Stiffness:** Morning stiffness or stiffness after periods of inactivity is a typical symptom. This stiffness normally improves with movement, but it may have a substantial impact on mobility and function, particularly in the morning or after sitting for an extended amount of time.

3. Swelling: The affected joints may seem swollen and heated to the touch. This swelling is caused by

inflammation and the buildup of synovial fluid in the joint area.

4. Reduced Range of Motion: As cartilage deteriorates and joint structures weaken, the afflicted joint's range of motion reduces. This constraint might impede everyday tasks and movement.

5. Crepitus is a grinding or crackling feeling that might occur when you move the joint. This is generally caused by the roughened surfaces of the joints grinding against one another.

6. Deformity: In severe instances, joint degeneration may cause noticeable abnormalities. For example, osteoarthritis in the hands may result in the growth of bone enlargements known as Heberden's and Bouchard's nodes.

Early detection of joint degeneration is critical for various reasons.

1. Preventing Further Damage: Early detection of joint degeneration allows for therapies to reduce the disease's development. Physical treatment, lifestyle changes, and medicines may help maintain residual cartilage and prevent additional damage.

2. Pain Management: Early diagnosis allows for timely pain management techniques, which improves the patient's quality of life. Effective pain treatment enables people to have an active lifestyle, which is essential for joint health.

3. Improving Function: Early treatments may enhance joint function and mobility, allowing people to do their everyday activities with more ease and less pain. Physical therapy and exercise regimes may help to strengthen the muscles around the joint, resulting in greater support and stability.

4. Avoiding Surgery: While joint replacement surgery is an excellent therapy for severe joint degeneration, early nonsurgical therapies may postpone or even eliminate the need for surgery. This lowers the dangers and recuperation times connected with surgical operations.

5. Better Long-Term Results: Patients who get an early diagnosis and adequate treatment are more likely to have positive long-term results. They can retain a greater degree of physical activity and independence, which is beneficial to general health and well-being.

How Does Joint Degeneration Affect Daily Life?

Joint degeneration may affect everyday living in a variety of ways:

1. Mobility Issues: Pain and stiffness might make walking, climbing stairs, or standing for long periods difficult. This may restrict involvement in jobs, social activities, and hobbies, lowering the overall quality of life.

2. Activity Restrictions: Joint degeneration often leads people to reduce or discontinue activities they previously loved. For example, a person with knee osteoarthritis may be unable to run or participate in sports, resulting in a more sedentary lifestyle and related health concerns.

3. Emotional Impact: Chronic pain and restricted movement may cause emotional and psychological problems. Many people feel frustrated, anxious, or depressed as a result of their restrictions and the ongoing suffering they face.

4. Independence Loss: Severe joint degeneration may make completing simple chores like dressing, bathing, and cooking difficult without help. This loss of freedom may be especially upsetting for those who treasure their autonomy.

5. Financial Burden: Managing joint degeneration may be expensive, requiring medical treatments, physical therapy, drugs, and perhaps surgery. Additionally, there may be indirect expenses associated with missed workdays and decreased productivity.

6. Sleep Disturbances: Pain and discomfort may disrupt sleep, resulting in exhaustion and poor overall health. Poor sleep quality exacerbates the impression of pain, potentially leading to a vicious cycle of pain and sleep disturbance.

Understanding joint degeneration, detecting symptoms early on, and seeking quick diagnosis and treatment may all help to improve the condition's management. Individuals may retain their quality of life and participate in their favorite activities by implementing suitable therapies and lifestyle adjustments.

CHAPTER 3

Preparing For Total Joint Replacement

Initial Discussions With Healthcare Professionals

The path to a successful total joint replacement starts with an in-depth consultation with healthcare professionals. This first step is critical in establishing the foundation for a well-informed and prepared surgery experience. During these discussions, many crucial actions occur:

1. Primary Care Physician Visit: Your primary care physician (PCP) will do a thorough examination of your general health. This involves a thorough medical history and physical examination. They will talk about your symptoms, the severity of your joint pain or dysfunction, and the effect on your everyday activities. To acquire preliminary data, your primary care physician may do basic diagnostic procedures such as blood tests and X-rays.

2. Referral to a Specialist: Based on the preliminary results, your PCP will recommend you to an orthopedic surgeon who specializes in joint replacement. The orthopedic surgeon will do a more detailed evaluation of the afflicted joint. They will examine imaging examinations such as X-rays, MRIs, and CT scans to establish the degree of joint damage and the need and feasibility of joint replacement.

3. Full Surgical Discussion: During your visit with an orthopedic specialist, you will be given a full description of the joint replacement surgery. This comprises the kind of joint replacement (e.g., hip, knee, shoulder), the materials utilized in the prosthesis, and the anticipated results. The surgeon will explain the risks, advantages, and consequences so that you know what to anticipate.

4. Questions and Concerns: Before meeting with your surgeon, make a list of your questions and concerns. Common questions include recovery time, pain management, physical therapy, and the prosthetic joint's lifetime. Addressing these questions can assist in reducing anxiety and increase trust in the surgical plan.

Medical Tests And Evaluations

Before having total joint replacement surgery, a battery of medical tests and examinations are performed to verify that you are in good condition for the operation. These tests are intended to discover any underlying disorders that may compromise surgery or recovery.

1. Blood tests are used to diagnose anemia, infections, and blood clotting abnormalities. These tests also provide information about your kidney and liver function, which is necessary for safe anesthetic delivery.

2. Imaging investigations: In addition to pre-consultation imaging, further imaging investigations may be necessary to provide a thorough understanding of the joint and surrounding structures. This allows the surgeon to design the exact placement of the prosthetic joint.

3. Cardiac Evaluation: Your heart's health is assessed using an electrocardiogram (EKG) and, in certain cases, a stress test. If you have a history of heart disease or are at risk, see a cardiologist.

4. Pulmonary Evaluation: A lung function test and chest X-ray are often done, particularly if you have a history of respiratory problems. This guarantees that your lungs are fit to withstand anesthesia and the demands of operation.

5. Preoperative Clearance: After all tests are done, your healthcare team will analyze the findings and grant preoperative clearance. If any problems are discovered, they will be rectified before continuing with surgery. This may include treating infections, regulating blood pressure, or controlling diabetes.

Lifestyle Modifications Before Surgery

Making lifestyle adjustments before surgery may greatly enhance your recovery and overall results. Here are some suggested changes:

1. **Weight Management:** If you are overweight, decreasing even a minor amount of weight may relieve joint tension and enhance surgery results. To help you attain a healthy weight, your healthcare professional might recommend a balanced diet and activity regimen.

2. **Exercise:** Following a specific exercise program may help to strengthen the muscles around the afflicted joint, enhancing stability and support. Low-impact activities such as swimming, cycling, and walking are often advised. Physical treatment may also be

recommended to improve your range of motion and muscular strength.

3. Smoking cessation: Smoking may slow recovery and increase the risk of complications including infections. It is best to stop smoking long before your operation date. Your healthcare practitioner may give you resources and assistance while you work to stop.

4. Alcohol use: Limiting or avoiding alcohol use before surgery is critical since it may interfere with anesthetic and postoperative drugs. Discuss with your healthcare physician the right steps to take about alcohol use.

5. Nutritional Supplements: Proper nutrition is essential for recuperation. Your doctor may offer iron, calcium, and vitamin supplements to help your immune system and bone health.

Mental And Emotional Preparations For Surgery

Preparing psychologically and emotionally for joint replacement surgery is as vital as physical preparation. Addressing your mental health issues may have a big impact on your recovery experience.

1. **Education and Expectations:** Understanding the whole procedure, from surgery to recuperation, helps create reasonable expectations. Attending pre-surgery courses, viewing instructional films, or reading information supplied by your healthcare team may be quite valuable.

2. **Worry Management Techniques:** Surgery may cause a lot of worry and anxiety. Deep breathing exercises, meditation, and mindfulness are all stress management practices that may help you remain calm and focused.

3. Creating a solid support system is critical. Inform relatives and friends about your surgery and recuperation requirements. Having someone to help with everyday tasks throughout your rehabilitation may make a big impact.

4. Counseling and Therapy: If you are experiencing severe anxiety or depression, consult with a mental health specialist. Counseling or therapy may provide coping methods and emotional support before and after surgery.

5. Journaling and Reflection: Writing down your ideas and feelings may help you process them and measure your development. Reflecting on your experience might help you feel motivated and accomplished while you heal.

By carefully preparing for total joint replacement, both physically and emotionally, you may improve your chances of a smooth operation and a quick recovery.

CHAPTER 4

Types Of Total Joint Replacement Surgery

Knee Replacement Surgery

An overview of surgery for knee replacement

Knee replacement surgery, also known as knee arthroplasty, is a popular treatment that involves To reduce discomfort and disability, the knee joint's weight-bearing surfaces are replaced. This operation is usually advised for those who have severe osteoarthritis, rheumatoid arthritis, or another kind of degenerative joint disease. The objective is to restore function and enhance quality of life.

Procedure Details

The operation entails removing diseased cartilage and bone from the knee joint's surface and replacing it with artificial metal and plastic components. This is how it's done:

1. The surgeon creates an incision above the knee to get access to the joint.

2. Knee joint resurfacing involves removing the damaged cartilage surfaces at the ends of the femur and tibia, as well as a tiny piece of underlying bone.

3. Positioning the Implants: Metal components are then positioned to reconstruct the joint surface. The underside of the kneecap is cut and resurfaced using a plastic button.

4. A medical-grade plastic spacer is put between the metal components to provide a smooth gliding surface.

5. The wound is closed with sutures or staples.

Recovery and Rehabilitation
Patients often spend a few days in the hospital after surgery. Physical treatment starts nearly immediately to promote mobility and strengthen the muscles that

surround the knee. Full recovery may take many months, and patients should follow an organized rehabilitation program to restore strength and mobility.

Hip Replacement Surgery

Overview of hip replacement surgery

Hip replacement surgery, also known as hip arthroplasty, involves replacing a diseased hip joint with a prosthetic implant. This surgery is often required because of disorders such as osteoarthritis, fractures, or other hip joint illnesses that cause discomfort and limit movement.

Procedure Details

The technique consists of many critical steps:

1. Incision and Joint Access: An incision is created over the hip to reveal the joint.

2. Removal of injured Bone and Cartilage: The injured femoral head is removed, and the hip socket surface is prepped.

3. Implanting the New Joint: A metal stem is placed into the femur. A metal or ceramic ball is used to replace the femoral head, which is then inserted into a metal socket lined with plastic or ceramic.

4. Reconstruction and closure: The replacement joint components are secured in place, and the incision is closed.

Recovery and Rehabilitation

Patients usually remain in the hospital for a few days after surgery. Early mobilization is recommended to avoid problems such as blood clots. Physical therapy is critical for restoring mobility and strength. Recovery might take months, with incremental improvements in walking and everyday activities.

Shoulder Replacement Surgery

Overview of Shoulder Replacement Surgery

Shoulder replacement surgery, also known as shoulder arthroplasty, involves replacing the shoulder joint with prosthetic components. This procedure is often used to treat severe arthritis, rotator cuff injuries, or fractures that impede shoulder function and create discomfort.

Procedure Details

The technique consists of the following steps:

1. Incision and Exposure: A cut is made above the shoulder to expose the joint.

2. Damaged Parts Removal: The humeral head is removed.

3. Implant placement: The humeral component (a metal ball) is joined to the residual bone, while the socket component is inserted into the shoulder blade.

4. Reconstruction and closure: The new components are attached, and the incision is closed.

Recovery and Rehabilitation

Patients spend a brief length of time in the hospital after surgery. Physical therapy begins shortly after to assist in recovering mobility and strength. Full recovery may take many months, with a focus on restoring range of motion and strength via an organized rehabilitation program.

Elbow Replacement Surgery

Overview of Elbow Replacement Surgery

Elbow replacement surgery, also known as elbow arthroplasty, is uncommon but essential for severe joint degeneration caused by illnesses such as rheumatoid arthritis, post-traumatic arthritis, or non-healing fractures. This procedure replaces the injured elbow joint with an artificial implant.

The steps are as follows:

1. An incision is made above the elbow to expose the joint.

2. Damaged joint surfaces are removed.

3. Implant placement: Metal and plastic components are utilized to replace joint surfaces. A hinge mechanism might be employed to connect the components.

4. Reconstruction and Closure: The new joint is stabilized, and the incision is closed.

Recovery and Rehabilitation

Recovery entails a hospital stay and quick post-operative physical treatment to avoid stiffness and regain mobility. Full recovery may take many months, with modest gains in strength and function achieved via a structured rehabilitation program.

Understanding these procedures, their processes and the recuperation period may help patients prepare for joint replacement surgery and establish reasonable expectations for the results.

CHAPTER 5

Surgical Procedure

Anesthesia Options

When having complete joint replacement surgery, selecting the right anesthetic is critical. There are two main types of anesthesia: general anesthesia and regional anesthesia.

General Anesthesia

General anesthesia is the process of putting the patient fully asleep during surgery. This approach assures that the patient is pain-free and unaware of the process. The anesthesiologist delivers the anesthetic medicines via an intravenous (IV) line or by inhaling via a mask. Once the patient is sleeping, a breathing tube is usually put in the windpipe to ensure appropriate breathing during the procedure.

Benefits Of General Anesthesia

• Ensures complete unconsciousness during operation.

• Provides a pain-free experience throughout the process.

• A controlled environment enables surgical teams to operate without patient mobility.

Drawbacks Of General Anesthesia

• Longer Recovery: Patients may have grogginess, nausea, and throat soreness after surgery.

• Potential complications from anesthesia include allergic reactions and respiratory issues.

Regional Anesthesia

Regional anesthesia numbs a particular region of the body, usually from the waist down, using spinal or epidural anesthesia.

The patient stays conscious but pain-free in the operative region. Sedatives may be used to assist the patient relax and sleep lightly throughout the treatment.

Benefits Of Regional Anesthesia

• Faster Recovery: Compared to general anesthesia, patients often wake up faster and with fewer side effects.

• Provides effective pain management during and after surgery, requiring fewer postoperative pain medicines.

• Lower chance of complications, including nausea and respiratory concerns, compared to general anesthesia.

Drawbacks Of Regional Anaesthesia

• Patient Awareness: Some patients may have anxiety about being awake during surgery, even if they do not feel pain.

- Patients may experience discomfort due to temporary loss of feeling and mobility in their lower body.

Choosing The Right Anesthesia

The patient's overall condition, medical history, and personal preferences all play a role in determining whether a general or regional anesthetic is used. The anesthesiologist will review these alternatives with the patient, taking into account any possible risks and advantages, to choose the best course of action for a safe and successful operation.

Surgical Techniques

Total joint replacement surgery employs a variety of procedures, each adapted to the exact joint being replaced and the patient's unique requirements. Here's a summary of typical surgical methods used in joint replacement procedures:

Traditional Open Surgery

Traditional open surgery is the most common type of joint replacement. It requires creating a big incision to have direct access to the joint. The surgeon removes the damaged joint surfaces and replaces them with prosthetic ones.

Steps For Traditional Open Surgery

1. A large incision is made to reveal the joint.

2. The surgeon gently removes the injured cartilage and bone.

3. Placement of Prosthetics: Metal, plastic, or ceramic components are placed and fastened.

4. Closure: Sutures or staples are used to seal the incision, followed by a sterile dressing.

Minimally Invasive Surgery

Minimally invasive surgery (MIS) uses tiny incisions and specialized equipment, resulting in less tissue damage. This approach may result in shorter recovery periods, less postoperative discomfort, and less scarring.

Steps For Minimally Invasive Surgery

1. Small Incisions: Incisions are generally just a few inches long.

2. Specialized Instruments: The surgeon utilizes specialized instruments to explore the joint and carry out the treatment via these microscopic incisions.

3. Prosthetic Placement: Similar to conventional surgery, prosthetic components are implanted via smaller incisions.

4. Close the minor incisions with sutures or staples.

Robotic Assisted Surgery

Robotic surgery uses modern robotic devices to improve accuracy. The surgeon directs the robotic arms, which can make very precise motions, often resulting in improved alignment and positioning of the prosthetic components.

Steps For Robotic-Assisted Surgery

1. Preoperative Planning: Detailed imaging scans are utilized to develop a surgical plan.

2. Robotic Assistance: During surgery, the robotic system aids with accurate motions and prosthesis implantation.

3. Incisions are formed, and robotic arms help to remove damaged tissue and place the prosthesis.

4. Closure: Incisions are closed in the same manner as in other surgical procedures.

Potential Risks And Complications

While total joint replacement surgery is typically safe and successful, patients should be informed of some risks and problems.

Infection

Infection is a dangerous complication that may develop at the incision site or deep into the new joint. Despite the use of preventative measures such as sterile methods and medications, infections may develop.

Signs Of Infection

• Fever: Increased body temperature.

• Increased redness, warmth, and swelling around the wound.

• Wound drainage may include pus or unusual discharge.

• discomfort: Unusual level of discomfort throughout mending.

Blood Clots

Blood clots, also known as deep vein thrombosis (DVT), may occur in the legs as a result of restricted movement after surgery. These clots may be harmful if they go to the lungs, resulting in a pulmonary embolism.

Prevention Of Blood Clot

• Medications: Blood thinners may be recommended.

• Use compression stockings or pneumatic compression devices.

• Early Mobilization: Encourages mobility and walking following surgery.

Prosthesis Issues

Prosthetic joint complications may include loosening, wear, or dislocation. These complications may need revision surgery.

Indicators of Prosthesis Problems

• Persistent discomfort in a joint region.

• Instability: Feeling the joint is unstable or giving way.

• Unusual noises from the joint, such as clicking or popping.

Nerve or Blood Vessel Damage

During surgery, there is a danger of injuring nearby nerves or blood vessels, resulting in numbness, weakness, or circulation difficulties.

Symptoms Of Nerve Or Vessel Damage

• Numbness refers to loss of feeling in the afflicted region.

• Weakness: Difficulty moving the joint and surrounding muscles.

• Circulation issues may include coldness, discoloration, or a lack of pulse in the extremities.

Expected outcomes

Total joint replacement surgery is intended to reduce pain, restore function, and enhance the quality of life for patients with significant joint injury. Understanding the anticipated results might assist patients in setting realistic objectives and planning for their recovery.

Pain Relief

One of the key advantages of joint replacement surgery is substantial pain alleviation. Most patients report a significant improvement in joint discomfort after the surgery.

Timeline of Pain Relief

• Medication is used to treat immediate post-surgery discomfort.

• First several weeks: Pain gradually decreases as the body recovers.

• Long-term relief from chronic pain caused by damaged joints.

Improved mobility

Improved joint function and mobility are important results. Patients may typically resume activities that were previously restricted due to joint discomfort and stiffness.

• Physical therapy is essential for recovering strength and flexibility.

• Slowly resuming regular activities with medical oversight.

• Long-term workouts help preserve joint function and avoid stiffness.

Patients often have a higher quality of life because of less pain and more mobility. They may engage in enjoyable activities while maintaining their freedom and improving their mental health.

• Easier to conduct daily activities such as walking, climbing stairs, and home duties.

• Ability to participate in leisure activities and sports.

• Improved pain management and independence lead to greater mental health.

The longevity of the prosthesis

Modern prosthetic joints are intended to survive for many years, often 15 to 20 years or more. However, its lifetime is dependent on variables such as activity level, weight, and adherence to postoperative care requirements.

Factors Influencing Prosthesis Longevity
• High-impact exercises may wear out joints quicker.

• Maintaining a healthy weight may lessen stress on joints.

• Regular check-ups with surgeons to monitor joint health.

Understanding these features of total joint replacement surgery enables patients to make more informed choices and prepares them for a successful surgical procedure and recovery.

CHAPTER 6

Recovery Process

Hospital Stay And Post-Operative Care

Following total joint replacement surgery, the recovery process often starts with a hospital stay. This time enables medical experts to carefully monitor your status and give any required postoperative care. The duration of your hospital stay depends on several variables, including the kind of joint replaced and your general health status.

During your hospital stay, you will get extensive postoperative care to ensure a smooth recovery. This involves monitoring vital signs, controlling pain, avoiding infections, and starting physical therapy as needed. Your medical team will constantly examine the surgery site for symptoms of problems, such as increased edema, redness, or discharge.

You'll also be coached through the early phases of therapy, which may include mild movements and exercises to improve blood circulation and reduce stiffness. It is critical that you carefully follow your healthcare provider's advice during this period to promote healing and reduce the chance of problems.

Once your medical team has determined that you are stable and suitable for release, you will be given instructions for at-home care and follow-up visits. These might include medication management, wound care instructions, and suggestions for progressively increasing exercise levels. To assist your recuperation and get the best possible results, you must strictly follow these recommendations.

Pain Management Strategies

Effective pain management is an important part of the rehabilitation process after total joint replacement surgery. While some discomfort is expected following surgery, proper pain management may help to reduce discomfort and improve recovery. Your medical team will create a pain management strategy tailored to your specific requirements and medical history.

Pain treatment techniques may use a variety of pharmaceuticals, such as over-the-counter pain relievers, prescription opioids, and nonsteroidal anti-inflammatory drugs (NSAIDs). These drugs assist in reducing pain and inflammation, enabling you to engage more easily in physical therapy and everyday activities.

In addition to drugs, your rehabilitation plan may include additional pain management approaches. Ice treatment, heat therapy, massage, acupuncture, and transcutaneous electrical nerve stimulation (TENS) are all possible options. These complimentary treatments may help decrease discomfort and improve relaxation, thus improving your entire healing experience.

It is important to discuss freely with your healthcare physician about your pain levels and any concerns you may have about pain treatment. Working together allows you to alter your pain management strategy as required to promote maximum comfort and healing throughout the rehabilitation process.

Physical Therapy And Rehabilitation

Physical therapy is essential in the rehabilitation process after complete joint replacement surgery. A comprehensive rehabilitation program customized to your unique requirements may help you regain mobility, strength, and function in the damaged joint. Physical therapy usually starts shortly after surgery and lasts for many weeks or months, depending on your progress.

During physical therapy sessions, you will engage with a qualified therapist who will lead you through a series of exercises and activities aimed at improving joint range of motion, muscular strength, and endurance. These exercises may include moderate stretching, strengthening exercises, balance training, and functional motions that are customized to your specific objectives and constraints.

In addition to in-person physical therapy sessions, you will get a home workout regimen to follow between visits. Consistently executing these exercises as instructed is critical to optimizing the advantages of physical therapy and attaining the best results. Your therapist will advise you on appropriate technique, progression, and safety concerns to ensure you exercise efficiently and safely.

As you proceed through physical therapy, you will progressively recover mobility and function in the replacement joint, enabling you to return to regular activities and improve your quality of life. To get the greatest outcomes, you must stay dedicated to your rehabilitation program and follow your therapist's suggestions.

Gradual Resumption Of Daily Activities

Returning to regular activities after total joint replacement surgery is a long process that involves patience, perseverance, and meticulous preparation. While you may be anxious to return to your usual routine, you must pace yourself and prioritize your health and safety throughout the recovery phase.

Your healthcare physician will advise you on when it is safe to resume particular activities depending on your personal development and the kind of joint replacement. You'll start with fundamental everyday tasks like walking, bathing, and dressing, then progressively increase the intensity and length of your activities over time.

It is important to listen to your body and avoid pushing yourself too hard, particularly during the first phases of rehabilitation. Pay attention to any indicators of weariness, discomfort, or joint pain, and modify your activity level appropriately. Remember that rest and good recovery are critical for helping your body to heal and adjust to the changes that occur after surgery.

As you develop strength, mobility, and confidence in your new joint, you will be able to progressively resume more strenuous activities including exercise, sports, and leisure interests. Your healthcare practitioner and physical therapist may advise you on how to proceed safely and prevent overexertion or injury during this transition phase.

You may improve your recovery and long-term results after total joint replacement surgery by taking a deliberate and organized approach to resume normal activities. Stay patient, and determined, and enjoy each milestone as you regain your mobility and freedom.

CHAPTER 7

Managing Expectations

Realistic Post-Surgical Expectations

When commencing on the road of total joint replacement, it is critical to have realistic expectations for the postoperative period. Understanding what to expect may help to make the healing process go more smoothly and increase overall happiness. While joint replacement surgery may significantly enhance mobility and quality of life, it is important to understand that it is neither a fast cure nor a guarantee of perfection.

Pain, edema, and stiffness in the operated joint are frequent symptoms immediately after surgery. This soreness is a normal component of the healing process and usually goes away gradually as time passes. However, expecting immediate alleviation or full restoration of function may result in disappointment and dissatisfaction. Instead, patients should expect modest recovery and set little goals along the way.

Rehabilitation is an important part of the healing process, and patients should be willing to commit to a full rehabilitation program recommended by their healthcare team. This program usually involves exercises to increase strength, flexibility, and range of motion in the afflicted joint. While these exercises may be difficult and unpleasant at first, they are necessary for restoring function and getting the most out of surgery.

Furthermore, it is critical to recognize that complete recuperation may take many months, and patience is required during this process. It is normal to have good and terrible days, and setbacks are an inevitable part of the road. Patients who retain an optimistic attitude and remain focused on long-term objectives may better traverse the ups and downs of rehabilitation.

Common Challenges During Recovery

Patients who have joint replacement surgery may face a variety of physical and mental obstacles throughout the recovery process. Understanding these problems may help people prepare psychologically and emotionally for the trip ahead, as well as devise solutions to overcome them.

Pain and discomfort management is a regular concern throughout the healing period. While pain medication may be administered to aid with discomfort, it is critical to strike a balance between pain treatment and the desire to be active and involved in rehabilitation. Finding the correct balance may need an open conversation with healthcare practitioners and changes to medication as required.

Another problem is recovering mobility and independence after surgery. Initially, patients may depend on assistive aids like crutches or walkers to go about securely.

As strength and mobility improve, these devices may be progressively taken away, but it is critical to proceed gently and follow the healthcare team's instructions to avoid falls or injury.

Patience and endurance are crucial traits throughout the rehabilitation process since improvement might be sluggish and gradual. It is natural to feel frustrated or doubtful at times, but keeping a good attitude and focusing on the final goal will help you overcome these obstacles. Furthermore, relying on the support of friends, family, and healthcare professionals may give important encouragement and drive during trying times.

Long-Term Advantages Of Joint Replacement

While the immediate advantages of joint replacement surgery are often seen in increased mobility and decreased pain, the long-term benefits go well beyond the first healing phase.

Joint replacement surgery, which addresses underlying joint degeneration and restores function, may dramatically improve quality of life and general well-being for many years.

One of the major long-term advantages of joint replacement is increased mobility and freedom. Individuals with better joint function may participate in activities that were previously restricted or difficult owing to pain and stiffness. Whether it's walking, hiking, gardening, or playing with grandkids, joint replacement surgery may lead to a more active and rewarding life.

Joint replacement surgery may help improve mental and emotional health. Chronic joint pain may hurt mental health, resulting in anxiety, despair, and a worse quality of life. Joint replacement surgery may restore a feeling of control and hope, enabling people to live their lives to the fullest.

Furthermore, joint replacement surgery may assist in preventing further joint deterioration and degeneration, thereby postponing or even eliminating the need for future surgical operations. Individuals who maintain a healthy weight, keep active, and follow a recommended fitness routine may extend the life of their joint replacements and get long-term advantages.

Lifestyle Changes For Improved Joint Health

Optimal joint health is critical for preserving mobility, independence, and general quality of life before and after joint replacement surgery. While surgery may treat current joint problems, maintaining a healthy lifestyle can help avoid additional degeneration and extend the life of joint replacements.

Maintaining a healthy weight is an important lifestyle modification for good joint health. Excess weight adds stress to the joints, especially weight-bearing joints like the knees and hips, increasing the risk of joint injury and degeneration. Individuals who achieve and maintain a healthy weight via a balanced diet and regular exercise may decrease joint strain and lower their risk of problems after joint replacement surgery.

Regular exercise is another important aspect of joint health, both before and after surgery. Low-impact exercises like swimming, cycling, and walking may assist increase joint flexibility, strength, and range of motion without putting too much strain on the joints. Furthermore, focused exercises given by a physical therapist may aid in the rehabilitation of the joint after surgery, preventing stiffness and muscle weakness.

In addition to nutrition and exercise, appropriate joint care includes avoiding behaviors that might worsen joint discomfort or injury. This might include high-impact exercises like sprinting or leaping, as well as repeated actions that impose undue pressure on the joints. Instead, people should prioritize activities that enhance joint health and general well-being while reducing the chance of injury.

Finally, emphasize rest and recovery to give the body time to mend and rebuild itself. Adequate sleep, stress management, and relaxation methods may all help improve joint health and general physical well-being. Individuals who take a holistic approach to joint care, which includes food, exercise, relaxation, and stress management, may optimize the advantages of joint replacement surgery and live a full and active lifestyle for many years.

CHAPTER 8

Complications And How To Handle Them

Infection Prevention And Management

One of the most important components of total joint replacement (TJR) surgery is infection prevention and control. Infection may arise at any point throughout the procedure, from pre-surgery preparation to post-operative care. To avoid infections, surgeons and healthcare personnel follow tight guidelines before, during, and after operations.

Patients may receive pre-operative tests to verify they are infection-free. This may involve blood testing, urine tests, and imaging scans to rule out any concealed infections. In addition, patients are often encouraged to wash with antibacterial soap the night before or morning of surgery to minimize the bacterial burden on their skin.

During surgery, the operating room is kept sterile, and the surgical team follows tight standards to reduce the risk of infection. Wearing clean gowns and gloves, using sterile devices and equipment, and utilizing procedures like antibiotic prophylaxis all help to lower the risk of infection.

Following surgery, patients are routinely examined for symptoms of infection, such as fever, redness, edema, or increasing discomfort at the surgical site. If an infection is suspected, diagnostic testing such as blood cultures or joint aspiration might be used to confirm the diagnosis.

If an infection is detected, immediate and urgent treatment is required to avoid future problems. This may include the use of antibiotics, either orally or intravenously, as well as surgical intervention to remove contaminated tissue or implants.

Blood Clot Prevention

Another possible side effect of TJR surgery is the development of blood clots, commonly known as deep vein thrombosis (DVT) or pulmonary embolism (PE). Blood clots may form when blood flow is limited, such as during surgery or lengthy periods of immobility after surgery.

Anticoagulant drugs may be given to patients before, during, and after surgery to help avoid blood clots. These drugs assist to thin the blood and prevent clots from forming. Furthermore, patients are often advised to walk and mobilize as soon as possible following surgery to enhance blood flow and lower the chance of clot formation.

Patients may also use compression stockings or pneumatic compression devices to promote circulation and avoid blood clots.

Despite these precautions, blood clots may still form, especially in individuals with specific risk factors, such as a history of clotting problems or extended immobility. Patients must be aware of the signs and symptoms of blood clots, such as swelling, discomfort, or warmth in the afflicted leg, and seek medical assistance as soon as they encounter any of these symptoms.

Implant Failure And Revision Surgery

While total joint replacement surgery is typically effective in relieving pain and improving function, there is always the possibility of implant failure or problems over time. Implant failure may be caused by a variety of causes, including wear and strain, loosening of implant components, and infection.

If an implant fails, revision surgery may be required to replace or repair any damaged components. Revision surgery is usually more involved and difficult than original joint replacement surgery since it may require removing scar tissue, treating bone loss, and choosing proper implants.

Before having revision surgery, patients will have a complete assessment to establish the reason for implant failure and the best next steps. This might involve diagnostic imaging tests like X-rays or CT scans, as well as meetings with orthopedic experts to discuss treatment choices.

Revision surgery is carried out with the same care and accuracy as the first joint replacement surgery, to restore function and alleviate discomfort. Depending on the intricacy of the modification, the recovery time may be longer and rehabilitation more extensive.

Psychological Support For Dealing With Complications

Patients may experience mental distress while dealing with problems after total joint replacement surgery. Pain, suffering, and the uncertainty of future surgery may all hurt mental health and well-being. As a result, psychological support is a vital component of overall treatment for patients having TJR surgery.

To assist patients deal with the physical and mental obstacles of surgery and recuperation, psychologists may provide counseling, support groups, or individual treatment. Furthermore, educating and informing patients about the surgical procedure, possible problems, and coping skills may help them feel more in charge of their recovery.

Healthcare practitioners play an important role in giving emotional support and assistance to patients throughout the surgical procedure. Healthcare staff may assist patients cope with the difficulties of TJR surgery by listening to their concerns, addressing their worries and anxieties, and giving comfort and encouragement.

In conclusion, difficulties after total joint replacement surgery are possible, but with adequate prevention, care, and support, patients may overcome these obstacles and obtain positive results. From infection control to psychological support, a holistic approach to treatment ensures that patients have the assistance and resources they need to negotiate the intricacies of TJR surgery and recover optimally.

CHAPTER 9

Living With Joint Replacements

Maintaining Joint Health Following Surgery

After joint replacement surgery, preserving the health of your new joint is an important part of your rehabilitation and long-term well-being. Your surgeon will offer particular advice based on your case, however there are some broad guidelines to follow.

First, strictly follow any specified drug schedule. This often includes pain medications and antibiotics to avoid infection. Pain management is especially crucial in the early stages of recovery since it improves mobility and participation in rehabilitation activities.

Second, adhere to the postoperative care requirements supplied by your healthcare staff. This may include wound care, physical therapy exercises, and limitations on some activities to protect the freshly replacement joint. It is critical that you talk freely with your healthcare professionals about any issues or problems you have during this time.

Another important part of preserving joint health following surgery is to emphasize relaxation and a good diet. Your body needs time to recuperate, so avoid overexertion and eat a healthy diet rich in key elements like protein, vitamins, and minerals. Proper hydration is essential for tissue healing and general health.

Additionally, be aware of your body mechanics and movement patterns to prevent putting undue strain on your new joint. This involves utilizing assistive equipment such as canes or walkers as necessary, as well as maintaining appropriate posture and body mechanics throughout everyday activities.

Finally, keep an eye out for any indicators of difficulties or problems with your joint replacement, such as increasing discomfort, swelling, or trouble moving about. Report any concerns to your healthcare physician right once to avoid problems and guarantee the best possible result from your operation.

Regular Follow-Up Appointments

After joint replacement surgery, frequent follow-up meetings with your surgeon are required to evaluate your progress and address any problems that may emerge. These sessions are often scheduled at regular intervals over the first year after surgery, gradually becoming less frequent as you recuperate.

During these sessions, your surgeon will assess your joint function, range of motion, and overall healing progress. They may also prescribe imaging tests, such as X-rays, to check the implant's integrity and identify any issues early on.

In addition to measuring your physical recovery, follow-up sessions allow you to address any obstacles or limits you are experiencing and change your treatment plan appropriately. As required, your surgeon may advise you to modify your exercise program, adjust your medication, or seek referrals to other healthcare providers such as physical therapists or pain management specialists.

Beyond the immediate post-operative period, monthly follow-up sessions are an essential part of long-term joint health maintenance. Your surgeon will check the status of your replacement joint over time and advise you on how to keep it functional and long-lasting.

As a patient, you should actively engage in these follow-up sessions by asking questions, noting changes in symptoms or function, and following any suggestions made by your healthcare team. By collaborating with your surgeon and other healthcare professionals, you may enhance the results of your joint replacement surgery and your quality of life.

Physical Activities And Exercises

Engaging in suitable physical activities and exercises is critical for optimizing the advantages of joint replacement surgery and preserving joint health over time. While it is critical to follow your surgeon's exact advice depending on your unique situation, there are some basic rules to keep in mind.

Low-impact activities like walking, swimming, and cycling are often suggested after joint replacement surgery because they promote cardiovascular health and muscular strength without putting too much stress on the replaced joint. These workouts may also assist in improving joint flexibility and range of motion, which promotes general function and mobility.

To maintain muscle tone and joint stability, in addition to aerobic activity, you should include strength training and flexibility exercises in your program. This may include workouts that target the muscles around the replacement joint, as well as stretching activities to increase joint mobility and reduce stiffness.

When participating in physical activities and exercises, it is important to listen to your body and avoid pushing yourself too hard, particularly in the early phases of recuperation. Begin carefully and gradually increase the intensity and length of your exercises as tolerated, taking note of any pain or discomfort.

It's also crucial to mix up your training program to avoid overuse problems and improve general health. Combining aerobic, weight training, and flexibility exercises may help you create a well-rounded fitness routine that benefits your joint health and general well-being.

Finally, before beginning any new fitness regimen, contact your healthcare professional, particularly if you have any underlying health issues or concerns. They may provide tailored suggestions and offer direction to help you safely and efficiently include physical activity in your post-operative rehabilitation plan.

Tips To Prevent Future Joint Problems

While joint replacement surgery may give great relief from pain and disability, it is critical to take proactive efforts to avoid future joint issues and extend the life of your restored joint. Here are some ideas to help you preserve joint health and function in the long run:

1. Maintain a Healthy Weight: Being overweight may put additional strain on your joints, causing them to wear out faster. Maintaining a healthy weight with a balanced diet and regular exercise will help you avoid future joint issues.

2. Stay Active: Regular physical exercise is critical for joint health and mobility. Low-impact workouts like walking, swimming, and cycling may help to strengthen muscles, increase flexibility, and maintain general joint function.

3. Protect Your Joints: Be aware of your body mechanics and movement patterns to prevent putting undue strain on your joints. To limit the risk of injury, use good lifting methods, avoid repeated activities, and wear supportive footwear.

4. Maintaining appropriate posture may assist transfer weight properly across your joints while also reducing strain on your muscles and ligaments. Pay attention to your posture when doing everyday tasks, and consider utilizing ergonomic supports or gadgets as necessary.

5. Avoid Overuse: Although physical exercise is beneficial to joint health, overuse may lead to joint inflammation and injury. Listen to your body and allow enough rest and recuperation time between sessions to avoid overuse problems.

6. Follow Up with Healthcare experts: Schedule frequent follow-up consultations with your surgeon and other healthcare experts to check the health of your replacement joint and address any concerns or difficulties that may occur. If you notice any new or worsening joint issues, get medical assistance right once.

By adopting these guidelines into your everyday routine, you may help safeguard your replacement joint and decrease the chance of future joint issues, giving you years of increased mobility and quality of life.

CHAPTER 10

Future Developments And Innovation

Advances In Joint Replacement Technology And Materials

In the field of joint replacement, technology, and materials play critical roles in improving patient outcomes and implant durability. Recent improvements have transformed the industry, providing more durability, usefulness, and biocompatibility.

One breakthrough is in the materials used in joint replacement implants. Traditional materials such as metal alloys and polymers have been augmented by newer, more durable alternatives such as ceramic composites and highly crosslinked polyethylene. These materials have greater wear resistance, which lowers the chance of implant failure and the necessity for revision operations. Furthermore, advances in surface coatings have improved osseointegration, resulting in greater implant durability and long-term success.

Furthermore, the introduction of computer-aided design and manufacturing (CAD/CAM) has improved the accuracy and personalization of joint replacement implants. Surgeons may now use patient-specific imaging data to design custom implants matched to individual anatomies, resulting in improved fit and alignment. This not only enhances surgical results but also reduces problems such as implant loosening and dislocation.

Furthermore, the use of robots and navigation systems in joint replacement procedures has improved surgical technique and precision. Robotic help enables more accurate bone excision and implant placement, decreasing intraoperative mistakes and increasing implant life. Furthermore, real-time navigation technologies provide surgeons with important input, assuring perfect placement and alignment during the treatment.

These technical innovations are always growing, providing even larger benefits in the future. From biocompatible nanomaterials to sophisticated imaging techniques, the landscape of joint replacement technology is ripe for future innovation, providing patients with increased functionality and lifetime.

Emerging Trends In Surgical Technique

Joint replacement surgical procedures have evolved significantly as a result of technological improvements, improved patient outcomes, and increased surgical experience. Emerging trends indicate a move toward minimally invasive treatments, quick recovery procedures, and patient-centered care.

Minimally invasive surgery (MIS) procedures have grown in popularity in recent years owing to their potential advantages, which include smaller incisions, less tissue stress, and quicker recovery. Using specialized devices and improved imaging modalities, surgeons may conduct joint replacement surgeries with more accuracy and less disturbance to the surrounding tissues. This leads to shorter hospital stays, less postoperative discomfort, and a faster return to functional activities for patients.

Furthermore, quick recovery techniques have evolved as a key component of contemporary joint replacement surgery. These procedures use a multidisciplinary approach, combining preoperative optimization, intraoperative approaches, and postoperative rehabilitation measures to accelerate recovery and reduce problems. Rapid recovery procedures aim to improve patient happiness and results while lowering healthcare costs by prioritizing early mobility, pain treatment, and patient education.

Another developing trend in surgical methods is the use of outpatient and ambulatory surgery facilities for joint replacement surgeries. Anesthesia, pain management, and surgical procedures have advanced to the point that joint replacement operations may be performed on the same day, enabling patients to go home the same day. This not only lowers healthcare costs but also increases patient convenience and happiness.

Furthermore, patient-centered care has emerged as a key component in the delivery of joint replacement therapies. Surgeons and healthcare professionals are increasingly integrating patient preferences, values, and objectives into treatment choices, which promotes collaborative decision-making and tailored care plans. By including patients as active partners in their treatment, healthcare practitioners may improve results and satisfaction while also increasing patient empowerment and autonomy.

As surgical methods progress, the future of joint replacement surgery promises even greater safety, effectiveness, and patient-centered care. From robotic-assisted surgeries to improved recuperation regimens, the landscape of joint replacement surgery is primed for further advancement, benefitting patients globally.

Research And Development In Regenerative Medicine

Regenerative medicine has enormous promise in the area of joint replacement since it provides fresh methods for tissue repair, regeneration, and function restoration. Recent research and development efforts have concentrated on leveraging the regenerative potential of stem cells, growth factors, and tissue engineering technologies to overcome the limits of conventional joint replacement procedures.

One area of investigation is the use of mesenchymal stem cells (MSCs) for tissue regeneration and repair. MSCs, which can differentiate into many cell types, show potential for improving healing and increasing tissue regeneration in injured joints. Clinical trials have investigated the use of MSC-based treatments for illnesses such as osteoarthritis, with encouraging findings showing improvements in pain, function, and joint integrity.

Growth factors such as platelet-rich plasma (PRP) have also received attention for their possible involvement in promoting tissue repair and regeneration. PRP, which is produced from a patient's blood, includes high quantities of growth factors that help speed up the healing process and reduce inflammation in damaged joints. Clinical trials have demonstrated that PRP injections may reduce pain and improve function in people with osteoarthritis and other joint problems.

Furthermore, breakthroughs in tissue engineering have resulted in the creation of biocompatible scaffolds and biomaterials for joint repair and regeneration. These scaffolds resemble the extracellular matrix found in joint tissues, creating a favorable environment for cell proliferation and tissue regeneration. Researchers want to produce bioengineered constructions that may restore damaged joint tissues while also retaining joint function by mixing biomaterials with cells and growth hormones.

While regenerative medicine shows enormous potential for the future of joint replacement treatment, important obstacles remain, such as refining cell delivery modalities, improving tissue integration, and assuring long-term safety and effectiveness. However, continuous research efforts are advancing our knowledge of regeneration mechanisms and refining therapeutic techniques, bringing us closer to developing regenerative therapeutics for joint problems.

Implications Of Future Innovations In Joint Replacement Therapy

The future of joint replacement treatment is being defined by continuous advances in technology, materials, and regenerative medicine, which have far-reaching consequences for patient care, results, and healthcare delivery. As these advances advance, numerous important implications arise for the area of joint replacement treatment.

One major impact is the possibility of individualized, precision medicine approaches to joint replacement. With advances in imaging, biomaterials, and computer modeling, surgeons may personalize treatment plans and implants to specific patient features, improving results and lowering problems. By incorporating patient-specific data such as anatomy, biomechanics, and genetics, doctors may provide genuinely individualized therapy that fits each patient's requirements and preferences.

Furthermore, future developments might usher in a paradigm shift toward regenerative therapy for joint problems. As our knowledge of stem cell biology, tissue engineering, and biomaterials grows, regenerative therapies have the potential to heal and restore damaged joint tissues, therefore postponing or even eliminating the need for standard joint replacement surgery. This has the potential to transform the management of illnesses like osteoarthritis by offering patients less intrusive, more long-lasting therapeutic alternatives that maintain joint function and quality of life.

Furthermore, advances in telemedicine and remote monitoring technology have the potential to revolutionize the delivery of joint replacement therapy. Patients may use telehealth platforms to get virtual consultations, preoperative education, and postoperative follow-up treatment from the comfort of their own homes. This not only increases patient convenience and accessibility but also allows for early intervention and continuity of treatment, resulting in better results and lower healthcare costs.

Finally, future developments in joint replacement treatment show enormous potential for increasing patient outcomes, improving surgical methods, and transforming joint disease care. From individualized implants to regenerative therapies and telemedicine alternatives, the future of joint replacement therapy promises significant breakthroughs for patients worldwide.

Conclusion

Finally, a thorough knowledge of total joint replacement (TJR) is critical for both patients and healthcare professionals. TJR, a surgical method used to restore function and relieve pain in patients with severe joint problems, is an important milestone in contemporary medicine. We have covered a wide range of topics in this book, from TJR indications and surgical procedures to post-operative care and possible problems.

One of the main lessons is the need for patient education and participation in decision-making. Patients seeking TJR should have a thorough grasp of their disease, the possible advantages and dangers of surgery, and reasonable expectations for the results. Furthermore, participating in pre-operative workouts and lifestyle changes may improve surgery results and assist in recuperation.

Surgical breakthroughs have resulted in improved implant designs, materials, and methods, leading to better functional results and longer joint replacement lifespans. However, it is critical to understand that TJR is not without dangers, such as infection, implant wear, and joint instability. Vigilant perioperative treatment and adherence to evidence-based guidelines are critical for reducing these risks and achieving positive results.

Post-operative rehabilitation is critical for regaining joint function and increasing patient independence. Physical therapy, occupational therapy, and home exercises are all essential components of the healing process, assisting patients in regaining strength, flexibility, and mobility. Furthermore, regular follow-up with healthcare specialists enables the early discovery and treatment of any difficulties or issues that may occur.

Beyond the clinical elements, TJR has a significant impact on patients' quality of life and general well-being. TJR allows people to resume everyday activities, engage in leisure activities, and live more active and meaningful lives by relieving pain and increasing joint function. Furthermore, the psychological benefits of TJR cannot be emphasized, as patients often report feelings of relief, pleasure, and empowerment after surgery.

In conclusion, complete joint replacement is an outstanding therapeutic strategy for those suffering from severe joint problems. TJR promises better function, less pain, and a higher quality of life via a multidisciplinary approach that includes patient education, surgical skills, and extensive rehabilitation. Moving ahead, ongoing research, innovation, and cooperation are critical to advancing the field of joint replacement and improving results for patients globally.

THE END

9 7 9 8 3 3 2 0 5 2 6 9 9